Common Chronic Illnesses and Their Treatments

A General Look at Common Health Disorders

By: James M. Lowrance © 2010

TABLE OF CONTENTS

INTRODUCTION:

This book is a collection of fourteen chapters addressing common health disorders, some which are also classified as chronic, inflammatory and/or autoimmune in nature. These illnesses have symptoms in-common with others that can manifest similarly and so a general understanding of them can help to distinguish them from other health disorders.

In addition to information regarding symptoms, I have also included general aspects regarding the diagnosis and treatment of these illnesses. It is my hope that the information contained in the chapters that follow is both informative and interesting for the listener. At the same time, it should be understood that proper diagnosis and treatment for any disorder affecting one's health, should be obtained through a medical professional.

NOTE: Chapter 14 covers two similar syndromes. These summaries of the health disorders covered in each chapter, are not intended to be extensive medical journals but rather contain the most important general information that most laypersons would be seeking on the subjects.

CHAPTER ONE

The Diagnosis and Treatment of Celiac Disease

The Autoimmune Disorder of Gluten Intolerance

Celiac Disease is an autoimmune condition of severe gluten intolerance that can cause digestive symptoms, malnutrition, anemia and damage to the digestive tract. Some medical sources are now of the opinion that "gluten sensitivity" can exist in patients, even when full-blown Celiac Disease is not present.

For some people, especially those who are already suffering from other autoimmune diseases; their bodies begin to develop intolerances to things they eat that contain wheat, barley, rye and oats (gluten and related proteins). Their bodies began to recognize these foods as being harmful and their immune systems create antibodies to attack cells found in the lining of the small intestine that help break down gluten so that the body absorbs the nutrients from it. As a result, inflammation develops in the digestive tract and the person suffering the condition will begin to experience symptoms.

The subheadings that follow below contain some basic facts on the symptoms, diagnosis and treatment of Celiac disease (also known as "Celiac sprue").

Symptoms of Celiac Disease

When intolerance to gluten triggers autoimmune reactions in the body, this is referred to as a food intolerance or allergy.

The symptoms may include the following.

• stomach pain

• diarrhea

• chronic indigestion

• nausea and vomiting

• hives/rash and itching

• mild fever

The symptoms vary among individuals affected and some people have very few symptoms while others may become quite ill. Over time, the disease can potentially result in permanent damage to the small intestine. People with long-term and severe cases, can also become deficient in necessary nutrients that can no longer be absorbed by the damaged small intestine. If left untreated, over time, this can result in anemia for some people and in weight loss, malnutrition and osteoporosis for others.

Blood Tests Help Diagnose Celiac Disease

When symptoms of gluten intolerance are identified in someone with Celiac disease, a doctor will order blood tests to detect the antibodies that cause the autoimmune response in the body. If the antibodies are positive, this usually provides a definitive diagnosis for the condition.

Some people however may test negative for the antibodies that cause Celiac disease but still suffer the disorder.

In these more rare cases, the doctor may order a biopsy to be done on the patient's small intestine. The tissue sample is then analyzed to determine whether the disease is present, so that proper treatment can be prescribed by a qualified physician.

Treatment for Celiac Disease

The most important part of treatment for Celiac disease is to remove all products containing gluten from the diet. This would include the following gluten-containing food products.

• oats

• wheat products

• breads

• cookies

• cereals

• beverages containing barely or malt

If inflammation in the small intestine is severe or not easily resolved by eliminating gluten from the diet, the treating doctor may prescribe a corticosteroid anti-inflammatory drug to reduce inflammation.

Treatment will also include supplementing the patient with any nutrients or vitamins that have become low in their system due to past or ongoing mal-absorption of them.

If damage to the small intestine occurs in a patient, medications to help with digestion and stomach upset may also be prescribed and rarely patients may need surgical removal of severely damaged areas of the small intestine.

If you experience allergy or intolerance to gluten food products, see your doctor for testing to determine if the cause is Celiac disease. If you suffer another autoimmune disease, this is even more important because it increases your risk for developing Celiac disease.

CHAPTER TWO

Diagnosing and Treating Sjogren's Syndrome

The Disease of Bodily Dryness

Sjogren's syndrome is an autoimmune, inflammatory disease that affects the fluid-producing and lubricating glands and tissues in the body.

Sjogren's syndrome (SS) can co-exist with other types of autoimmune diseases and is especially common in people who suffer autoimmune thyroid diseases and rheumatoid arthritis. The severity of the disease varies among patients who have it and in some cases, it can become disabling. There are however, treatments available that can lessen the effects of symptoms and in some cases reverse them into near-remission.

Sjogren's Syndrome Dries-Out the Body

Sjogren's syndrome (pronounced "show-grins") affects the fluid producing ducts and glands of the body, as well as mucous membranes in the body. When a person has SS, the immune system has sent out killer cells, called antibodies, to attack these mechanisms of the body that produce lubricating fluids and membranes. This, results in these fluids and membranes becoming dry, so that the parts of the body that contain them may also become inflamed.

The areas of the body that can be affected by SS include:

- the tear ducts in the eyes
- the saliva ducts under the tongue
- the sinuses
- the skin
- the digestive system
- in women, the vagina is also commonly affected

Some patients are affected in only one or two areas of the body, such as the mouth or eyes, but the disease can also become systemic (body-wide).

Symptoms of Sjogren's Syndrome

In addition to patients experiencing dryness in the parts of the body listed above, SS can also result in fatigue, joint pain, digestive problems, skin rashes, muscle weakness, dental cavities and neuropathies (nervous system symptoms). In fact, SS can affect any organ in the body if it is chronic and severe, including the blood vessels. People with SS also tend to develop lung infections more easily. Cold and flu viruses will often result in bronchitis.

Diagnosing Sjogren's Syndrome

In addition to the symptoms that lead a doctor to suspect Sjogren's syndrome, there are also blood tests that help to detect SS and other medical tests that can lead to a diagnosis.

These blood tests include ones to detect antibodies that cause the autoimmune disease, referred to as the "SSA and SSB" antibodies tests.

Doctors may also order blood tests to detect systemic auto-antibodies, referred to as the Antinuclear Antibodies or the "ANA." A blood test for inflammation may also be ordered, called the "ESR," which helps to detect inflammatory reactions that might be present in the body. Some patients who have SS in more localized areas of the body may test negative, yet still have the disease.

For patients suspected of having SS affecting the mouth, some doctors will have a biopsy performed on saliva gland tissue. A special type of absorbent paper may also be used to test patients whose eyes are specifically affected. The paper is placed on the tear ducts of the eyes and the amount of tear fluid can be observed to see if inadequate amounts are being produced.

Treatment for Sjogren's Syndrome

There is no specific treatment for this autoimmune disease and so the treatment is to reduce the effects of the bodily symptoms it causes. For patients who experience dry eyes, doctors may prescribe synthetic tear solutions or pharmaceutical grade eye drops to help keep the eyes lubricated.

The same is true of patients with dry sinuses; nose drops may be prescribed to help moisturize the dry tissues in the nose and sinus passages.

Patients with joint pain may be prescribed medications to treat arthritic and rheumatic symptoms. For those patients with chronic and severe inflammation, a corticosteroid may be prescribed to reduce the inflammation, such as the commonly prescribed anti-inflammatory called "Prednisone."

Patients who are experiencing the previously-described symptoms should consult with their physician, to see if he recommends testing for Sjogren's syndrome. This is especially true in patients who are already experiencing other autoimmune diseases.

CHAPTER THREE

Diagnosing and Treating Pernicious Anemia

Tired Blood from Low B12 Levels

Symptoms of pernicious anemia, caused by low vitamin B12 are those of other types of anemia, with the addition of neurological symptoms that can occur in severe cases.

All conditions of anemia result in low or inadequate red blood cell counts, causing patients to have tired blood. This simply means that the red blood cells are inadequate to carry sufficient amounts of oxygen to the tissues of the body for energy. This is true of pernicious anemia as well, a condition resulting from low levels of vitamin B12.

Symptoms of Anemia

The general symptoms of anemia from low B12 and other causes may include the following.

• weakness and fatigue

• headache

• dizziness

• pale complexion

• fast heartbeat (tachycardia)

• shortness of breath

• difficulty concentrating

• cold extremities

People with pernicious anemia are also at risk for developing neurological symptoms if the condition worsens due to treatment-delay or non-treatment. These more advanced symptoms may include the following.

• numbness, burning and/or tingling in the legs, arms, feet and hands

• loss of muscle coordination and muscle weakness

• ringing in the ears

• dizziness and loss of balance

• slowed or erratic reflexes

• irritability, confusion, anxiety and depression.

The Cause of Pernicious Anemia

Pernicious anemia is specifically caused by vitamin B12 deficiency. Vitamin B12 is an important vitamin that plays an essential role in the development of red blood cells. In some countries where diets are inadequate due to low intake of foods rich in vitamin B12, such as liver, red meats, poultry and dairy products, there is a higher risk for the development of pernicious anemia.

The low state of vitamin B12 is often caused by an autoimmune process in industrialized countries, while poor diet is a less common cause.

The highest percent of cases in the USA and the UK for example, are caused by this autoimmune process, whereby the immune system turns on a natural substance in the digestive system called "intrinsic factor" and destroys it, rendering it incapable of absorbing proper amounts of vitamin B12 from foods eaten.

When Intrinsic Factor Becomes Deficient

This essential B12 vitamin is absorbed by the body from foods, through the digestive system via intrinsic factor, which is a protein that allows for this absorption process to take place. In some people, especially those who have autoimmune diseases, the body will begin to create "antibodies" (killer cells from the immune system), directed against intrinsic factor. Over time, these antibodies begin to destroy this substance and the body will eventually have inadequate amounts available (deficiency) for absorbing vitamin B12 from the diet.

People who already have disorders – such as autoimmune thyroid disease, celiac disease, Crohn's disease, Addison's disease (adrenal glands), lupus, rheumatoid arthritis and other autoimmune disorders – are at higher risk for developing pernicious anemia.

Treatment for Pernicious Anemia

Pernicious anemia is treated by replacing the low vitamin B12 level. When a doctor confirms that a person has become anemic, blood tests for the cause of the anemia will then be conducted.

If the cause is found to be low B12 levels, the treatment prescribed will be to replace the low vitamin to get it back to a normal level, via one or more of the methods described as follows.

• Vitamin B12 injections to replenish low levels, administered on a regular schedule, such as once-monthly, usually lifelong.

• Oral B12 in the form of tablets or liquid, as long as patients do not have sensitivity (side effects) to the oral form of the vitamin.

• Iron supplements administered to patients needing it in addition to replacement of low B12 levels.

It was once believed that injections were the only method of B12 replacement for severe deficiencies, but recent medical research articles published on the PubMed (U.S. National Institutes of Health) medical research website state that oral B12 in sufficiently high amounts can successfully treat B12 deficiency.

Diagnosing Pernicious Anemia

Blood testing of the B-12 levels is the most definitive test for pernicious anemia. Anemia can be confirmed through a "Complete Blood Count" blood test (CBC), but the test that definitively diagnoses pernicious anemia is a blood test of the vitamin B-12 level. Blood testing labs have normal ranges/values that vary, but if a lab has for example, a normal range for vitamin B-12 of between "200 to 1200 pg/ml" and the patient's result is "150 pg/ml" this would indicate B-12 deficiency as the cause of the anemia.

There is also a blood test to detect antibodies against the protein called intrinsic factor, and if this test comes back positive for these antibodies, this will reveal to the patient and to their doctor that the pernicious anemia is caused by an autoimmune process.

Pernicious anemia is an autoimmune disorder and is more common in patients who already suffer from other types of autoimmune diseases. The preceding subheadings can help one to recognize and understand treatment methods for this potentially serious type of anemia caused by vitamin B12 deficiency.

CHAPTER FOUR

Acid Reflux and Lung Disorders

GERD and Respiratory Illnesses

Gastroesophageal Reflux Disease (GERD) is a common cause of breathing problems, including bronchitis, asthma and pneumonia.

GERD can be a direct trigger for these pulmonary (lung) disorders or can worsen them in people with an already existing breathing problem. This occurs due to acid from the stomach, making its way into the windpipe and/or breathing tubes of the lungs. There are treatments available for the acid reflux that can lead to these respiratory problems.

What is GERD?

Gastroesophageal Reflux Disease is a condition in which contents in the stomach, such as food, liquids and stomach-acid travel up into the esophagus causing a heartburn sensation. The esophagus is the tube that goes from the mouth down to the stomach and there is an upper valve that closes it off from the windpipe with swallowing (the sphincter) to prevent food from being inhaled.

What Causes GERD?

GERD can occur over time with consuming spicy and/or foods or with eating very large meals.

It can be aggravated by eating too close to bedtime, in which the full stomach has not had time to fully digest its contents (indigestion). It can also manifest more severely with excess weight in the mid section, which adds pressure on the stomach, especially when laying flat on one's back.

The typical symptoms of GERD may include the following.

• heart burn

• sour stomach

• bitter flavor in the mouth

• mild chest pain

• an urge to swallow often

• a sensation of food moving upward into the throat

How GERD Affects Breathing

While food may not make its way into the windpipe when acid reflux occurs, stomach acid may still irritate the upper portion of the esophagus and the opening of the windpipe. Over time, very small amounts of stomach acid will seep into the lungs, causing irritation of the breathing passages in the lungs (bronchial tubes). Some GERD sufferers can experience episodes of actually choking on stomach acid and/or food particles that make their way into the breathing tube.

Symptoms of a breathing problem can include the following.

• coughing

• wheezing

• popping or crackling sounds when breathing

• uncomfortable feeling in the chest (usually tightness)

• shortness of breath with mild exertion

Resulting Breathing Disorders

A common breathing problem that can result from GERD is bronchitis, which is a term simply meaning that the bronchial tubes have become irritated and inflamed which often causes them to become congested. Some cases of bronchitis first manifest with a dry cough (non-productive) and afterward, the lungs will begin to secrete mucous (phlegm) in an attempt to push out bacteria and inflammation. At this point, the cough becomes productive (or may start out productive). The phlegm will often remain as a clear-colored non-infectious type that clears-up over an approximate two week period.

In more severe cases of bronchitis, the phlegm may develop into a white, green or yellow color or have streaks of blood found in it, which can indicate developing pneumonia or chronic bronchitis (ongoing).

These are more serious forms of infectious lung illness that can cause permanent lung damage and scarring and may contribute to COPD (Chronic Obstructive Pulmonary Disease). It can also become an emergency situation and can require hospitalization due to the extreme difficulty in breathing that can result.

Asthma is also a common finding in GERD patients and this condition simply indicates that the bronchial tubes in the lungs are constricting, causing difficulty with breathing. Cases of asthma can be mild, moderate or severe. This constriction within the lungs in cases of GERD is the body's attempt to prevent more food particles or acid from entering into them. Sometimes bronchitis and asthma occur together, which is referred to as "bronchial asthma."

Treatments for Acid Reflux

Research studies have shown that 75% of people with chronic cough from bronchitis and/or asthma will improve with treatment of co-morbid (co-occurring) GERD. Treatments may include over-the-counter antacids, prescription acid blocker medications (H2-blockers) and lifestyle changes.

Doctors will often recommend that patients lose excess weight and eat lighter meals that are not spicy. They may also recommend that GERD patients elevate the head of their beds a few inches, which helps to keep acid from rising into the throat.

Patients should eat their evening meals no closer than three hours before bedtime.

Severe damage (erosion) of the esophagus can result in the need for surgical repair and some cases of GERD develop into a condition called "Barrett's Esophagus", a pre-cancerous condition that may require removal of a section of the esophagus.

While actual breathing disorders require separate treatments of their own, treating GERD can help to prevent these illnesses from developing and help patients to recover or improve from existing breathing disorders.

CHAPTER FIVE

Rheumatoid Arthritis Basic Facts

Autoimmune Joint Disease

Statistics state that approximately 2.1 million Americans are affected by rheumatoid arthritis (RA) and it is more common in people who suffer other autoimmune diseases.

This form of arthritis causes destruction of the joints over time if treatment is not administered and in some cases can also cause joints to become locked in place (fused) and immobile. While RA has no cure, there are treatments that can place the disease in near-remission or significantly slow its progression. It typically affects the small joints in the extremities (hands and feet) but can potentially affect any of the joints of the body.

RA is an Autoimmune Disease

In the case of RA, the immune system recognizes components involving the areas of the body where bones attach to each other (joints) as threats in the body and sends out killer cells called "antibodies" to attack them. These natural body tissues are mistakenly identified by the immune system as intruders or invaders that threaten bodily health.

The joint-related tissues affected include the following:

- bones

- cartilage

- fibrous tissue

- synovial fluid

Medical science has yet to identify singular, specific causes for why autoimmune diseases occur but research continues in this area.

Symptoms of RA

As with other types of arthritis, joint pain and stiffness are major symptoms of RA but because the condition is autoimmune and not simply a natural wearing-away of bones and cartilage from the continual use or overuse of them (osteoarthritis), other symptoms will also manifest. These may include the following:

- redness and swelling around joints

- symmetrical manifestation – both sides of the body equally affected

- fever

- fatigue

- anemia due to loss of red blood cells

- loss of appetite

Diagnosing RA

In addition to recognizing the symptoms that point to a patient having RA, a doctor may also order the following blood tests to diagnose the disease

- RA Factor
- Anti-Nuclear Antibodies (ANA)
- Erythrocyte Sedimentation Rate (ESR)

The RA Factor and ANA tests are designed to detect levels of antibodies that cause the disease while the ESR test is designed to detect high levels of inflammation in the body. Some patients may not test positive for antibodies and/or an elevated ESR but may still be diagnosed based on physical symptoms that are present.

Treatments for RA

The goal for treating autoimmune arthritis is to control and alleviate symptoms being experienced and to slow the progression of the disease to prevent joint destruction, unnatural bone fusions and deformities.

Patients with less severe inflammation may be prescribed milder types of anti-inflammatory drugs such as ibuprofen, indomethacin or naproxen. In more severe cases, prescription-strength anti-inflammatory medications may be required called "corticosteroids".

These are steroids that mimic the inflammation moderating properties of the adrenal hormone "cortisol."

Less common treatments used to treat more progressed cases of RA include the injection of "gold compounds" into the joints and imunno-suppressive drug therapies to slow-down over activity by the immune system. Additional drug therapies that may be used in some cases may include D-penicillamine, anti-malarial drugs, and sulfasalazine.

With proper treatment, most RA patients can resume a relatively normal level of physical activities and an improved quality of life.

CHAPTER SIX

Metabolic Syndrome Basic Facts

The Condition of Metabolism Dysfunction

Metabolic Syndrome (METS) affects an estimated 25% of Americans in-general with people age 50 and above being the most affected (44% in this age group).

METS, formerly known as "Syndrome X," is a pre-diabetic condition that can affect blood pressure, cholesterol levels, glucose and triglyceride levels and weight gain. It also causes the body to become resistant to the pancreatic, glucose-regulating hormone "insulin" (insulin resistance). If not treated, the syndrome increases the risk for development of diabetes and heart disease. For those who already have diabetes, the condition is commonly co-morbid (co-occurring). It also occurs more commonly in patients with other endocrine disorders including thyroid disease.

Symptoms of METS

Physical symptoms are either non-existent or vague and can include the following:

• weight gain

• fatigue

• exercise intolerance

• increased hunger and thirst

• frequent urination

• hypoglycemic or hyperglycemic episodes (sudden drop or rise in blood glucose)

The symptoms experienced are similar to those of diabetes but are typically milder and may be intermittent or more noticeable at nighttime.

Hypertension (high blood pressure) is common with METS but is a symptom that does not typically cause physical sensations in the body and is usually found incidentally with a blood pressure monitor. The same is true of the elevated total-cholesterol, glucose and triglyceride levels it may also cause, which can only be detected by blood lab testing. The results will usually reveal elevated LDL cholesterol (unhealthy type) and an HDL cholesterol level (healthy type) that is flagged low. Fasting glucose and triglyceride levels will often be flagged high with the syndrome as well.

Causes of METS

A major cause of the syndrome is obesity, especially the type that affects the mid-section of the body (waistline). Men, whose weight gain results in a waistline that is 40-inches or greater in circumference and women whose weight gain results in a 35-inch waistline or greater, are at high risk for the onset of METS.

Lack of proper exercise is also a major contributing factor.

When physical activity slows down to an abnormally low level, less fat is being converted by the body into energy and will instead be stored in the body. This results in weight gain, hypertension, elevated cholesterol and an increase in blood glucose.

Improper diet can also contribute to the onset of METS. This would be a diet lacking the proper types of healthy carbohydrates and proteins but instead consists of an overabundance of fatty and sugary foods.

Treatments for METS

A healthy diet should be implemented that contains servings of the following foods:

• fruits

• vegetables

• nuts

• grains

• chicken and lean meats

These are "complex carbohydrates" rich in protein and fiber.

The diet should not consist largely of "simple carbohydrates" but very little or none, which include the following junk foods and drinks:

• soft drinks

• candy

- pies

- cookies

- cakes

- alcohol

The body will very quickly convert these "junk foods" into energy which causes a craving for more of them. This is due to the body's need for a steady energy-level which can be instead provided by the healthy foods previously listed. Weight loss should also be a priority. This can be accomplished by eating the proper foods previously listed and by eliminating the unhealthy ones containing simple carbohydrates and refined sugars (those not occurring naturally).

Getting proper exercise, especially the aerobic type, can also aid in weight loss but can also help regulate glucose and cholesterol levels by helping the body to burn fat and glucose into energy. It is important however that any exercise regimen is carefully practiced to make sure the body's tolerance level for it is not exceeded.

Patients with METS should discuss treatment with their doctor that is best tailored to their individual needs and that may include prescription drugs to control hypertension, insulin resistance and/or elevated glucose levels.

A doctor can also refer patients who smoke to non-smoking programs or drugs to help them quit.

CHAPTER SEVEN

Systemic Lupus Erythematosus Basic Facts

An Autoimmune Connective-Tissue Disease

There are basically four types of lupus erythematosus (LE). The disease is also considered to be of the inflammatory and rheumatic type.

Types of lupus erythematosus (LE) include "discoid" (round lesions and scarring affecting the skin), "neonatal" (present at birth), "drug-induced" (resulting from illegal drug-use or prescription ones) and "systemic" (multi-organ, tissues, blood vessels and cells). Patients diagnosed with discoid LE, are at high risk for developing the systemic type. Many patients with LE go on to develop other autoimmune diseases as well, such as those affecting endocrine glands (i.e. thyroid, pancreas and adrenals) and rheumatoid arthritis.

Who is Affected by LE?

The disease affects approximately one million Americans, with about 90% of those patients being women. Research published by the U.S. National Institute of Arthritis and Musculoskeletal and Skin Diseases (NIAMS) states that African American women are at higher risk for developing the disease. Approximately 1 in 250 black women will contract the disease by early adulthood.

It is also more common in Hispanic Asian and Native American women than in Caucasians.

Auto-antibodies and Inflammation

For reasons yet to be fully determined by medical research, the body will turn against itself with autoimmune diseases, resulting in the creation of auto-antibodies that begin to attack natural tissues, organs or cells in the body. With LE, the organs that are attacked can include the kidneys, lungs, skin, blood vessels (vasculitis) and blood cells (hemolytic anemia).

In addition to these specific antibodies, the disease is also characterized by "anti-nuclear antibodies" (ANA) that indicate systemic autoimmunity occurring in the body. If these antibodies are found to be positive when they are blood-tested for, this can help to diagnose LE.

The disease causes systemic inflammation in the body, rather than localized inflammation such as that found in autoimmune thyroid diseases for example, which usually cause limited inflammation. Another blood test called the Erythrocyte Sedimentation Rate (ESR) can help to detect high levels of inflammation in the body caused by LE.

Symptoms

One major characteristic symptom of systemic LE is a butterfly shaped rash on the face that appears on the cheeks, nose and forehead.

Other symptoms may include:

• Chronic Fatigue

• Joint and muscle pain and weakness

• Severe rashes on various part of the body that may be worsened by sun exposure

• Irregular menses (periods)

• Changes in body weight (loss or gain)

• Dry eyes and skin

• Hair loss or brittleness

• Fever

• Loss of blood circulation to hands and/or feet and discoloration in them (Raynaud's phenomenon)

• Hormone imbalances

Symptoms vary among patients, depending on how advanced a case of LE is and which organs are being affected.

Treatment

While there is no cure for LE, there are treatments designed to help relieve symptoms and to slow or halt the progression of the disease. Anti-inflammatory drugs may be recommended or prescribed depending on the strength needed. Some patients may only need over-the-counter drugs for inflammation and/or fever, such as aspirin or ibuprofen.

Others may need those that are prescription-strength anti-inflammatory steroids (corticosteroids).

Drugs that help to control immune system activity may also be prescribed as well as pain medications and hormone replacement therapies when needed. People, who believe they may be experiencing symptoms indicating LE, should see a licensed medical doctor as soon as possible.

CHAPTER EIGHT

Non-Alcoholic Fatty Liver Disease and NASH

Fatty Infiltration of the Liver and Steatohepatitis

Fatty liver disease that is non-alcohol related is very common, affecting up to 30% of the general population and is associated with obesity and endocrine disorders.

Non-Alcoholic Fatty Liver Disease (NAFLD - steatosis) is a condition in which an abnormally high number of cells in the liver become infiltrated with fat. Non-Alcoholic Steatohepatitis (NASH) is a more serious version of the condition, in which inflammation and possible liver damage develops in addition to fatty infiltration. While most cases of NAFLD do not develop into the more serious NASH stage of the disease, it is important for those who are diagnosed, to be monitored regularly for any signs of significant disease-progression. Even when NASH does develop, it does not lead to liver damage in most cases but increases the importance in the condition being monitoring by a qualified physician.

NAFLD and NASH Symptoms and Blood Lab Results

Most patients do not experience symptoms with NAFLD and the condition is often found incidentally when blood tests are run and the condition shows up on liver function tests.

The liver enzymes that are included on liver-panel lab tests include the ALT (alanine aminotransferase) and the AST (glutamic-oxaloacetic transaminase), both of which can detect liver damage from very mild to severe, depending on how highly elevated above normal values they become. Typical cases of NAFLD, present with mild to moderate elevations of liver enzymes while NASH will often present with very high elevations. NASH patients are also observed for the presence of any physical symptoms that might indicate serious liver disease, such as jaundice (yellowing of the skin and/or eyes), dark colored urine and pain or swelling on the right side of the abdomen, just below the ribcage.

Confirming with Liver Ultrasound

Once abnormal liver enzyme counts are discovered and/or any physical symptoms of possible liver problems, a treating doctor will often refer the patient to a radiology lab technician to have a liver ultrasound performed. This test uses highly sensitive sound waves to transmit an image on a monitoring screen, to look for any abnormal textures, stones or lesions (damage) in the liver. The test also detects fatty infiltration of the liver, which will cause the organ to appear glossy in texture on the surface, which is referred to as an abnormal echogenicity. This type finding helps to confirm blood test results that point to NAFLD.

Liver Biopsy

If liver ultrasound does not reveal lesions, stones or damaged areas on the liver, no further testing is usually done. If however, the liver appears to have these type problems or other findings such as tumorous growths, an additional test, taking a tissue sample of the liver to be further analyzed might also be ordered. This is usually done using a hypodermic needle that is of the correct length, to insert into the liver from the surface of the skin while a patient is under anesthesia. A biopsy can detect malignancy (cancer cells), as well as irreversible liver damage which is referred to as cirrhosis (scarring).

Treatment for NAFLD and NASH

Patients diagnosed with NAFLD, will be given the recommendation to lose any excess weight and to modify their diets to reduce fatty foods and refined sugars, which can also convert into fat cells. Unhealthy fats that can cause problems including fatty liver and elevated cholesterol are called trans-fats and include hydrogenated and partially hydrogenated oils found in fried foods and simple carbohydrates (junk foods). Increasing intake of foods with fiber is also a common recommendation because it helps to clear the body and liver of excess stored fats.

Healthy foods that help rid the body of unhealthy fats include fruits, vegetables, nuts and grains.

Even though NAFLD is not caused by alcohol consumption, patients are also advised not to drink alcohol due to its potential damaging effect on the liver. Regular exercise to a patient's tolerance level may also be recommended due to its many benefits including burning fat cells into energy. If a patient has co-existing diabetes, insulin resistance or thyroid disease, keeping these other metabolic-related disorders well-treated can also help. NASH patients will be given the same diet and lifestyle recommendations but may also be treated with additional drug therapies such as insulin-sensitizing agents and other drugs typically used to treat diabetes. Medical research continues in attempting to find effective drugs and supplements (including studies of vitamin E) for treating NASH.

CHAPTER NINE

Thyroid Autoimmunity

Autoimmune Diseases of the Thyroid Gland

Autoimmune thyroid disease is the most common of all autoimmune diseases. Thyroid diseases in general affect an estimated 27- million Americans, 80% of those having the type causing "hypothyroidism" and are five to eight times more common in women than in men (statistics vary).

The majority of thyroid disorders are caused by autoimmune disease and result in either an under-functioning thyroid (HYPO-thyroidism) or an over-functioning thyroid (HYPER- thyroidism). The symptoms of each of these can be severe and very concerning to the person experiencing them. With hypothyroidism the thyroid gland is slowed down in its ability to produce and distribute "thyroid hormone", which are the cells designed to control the metabolism in our entire body. So the thyroid, in a sense, is like a thermostat that regulates the rate at which our bodies operate at. With hyperthyroidism the thyroid gland is sped up, producing and distributing too much thyroid hormone. As stated before, both of these are most commonly caused by autoimmune disease of the gland.

Autoimmune disease is an improper response by our own immune system.

It should normally only direct this response against viruses, allergies, fungus and bacteria but at times, for reasons yet understood by medical science, it will direct this response against normal cells or organs, as if they are one of these intruders/invaders. The immune system does this by sending killer-cells called "antibodies" that literally attack and kill these unwanted enemies of our bodies. If these antibodies begin attacking an organ, such as the thyroid gland, they will relentlessly do so, until they cause damage to the gland and it begins to malfunction.

When you have thyroid autoimmunity, this can cause illness, apart from thyroid hormone levels. This is a fact that many Doctors do not seem to recognize because they are of the opinion that until the disease actually lowers or raises hormone levels to abnormal levels, patients will have no symptoms from the disease.

First of all, the thyroid autoimmunity, of itself, causes inflammation in the body. It can also cause goiters and nodules in patients who have normal thyroid hormone levels. Thyroid autoimmunity also causes other illnesses, as stated in reputable research articles. The ill feeling patients get with thyroid disease, is in part due to the disease itself.

Some patients with highly elevated antibodies may feel ill even when they are on proper thyroid dose.

They may need an anti-inflammatory or supplements like selenium, to help lower the antibodies and their effects. Their thyroid medications over time will also help do this.

There are many research articles, stating the same conclusions, that the thyroid autoimmunity itself is a cause of symptoms. These conclusions, from research conducted over a span of many years, is still unknown or unrecognized by many Doctors. The articles contain such phrases as; "systemic inflammatory reaction", caused by thyroiditis. This means the inflammation is not always localized, only in the area of the thyroid as some Doctors will tell their patients.

My belief is that some patients have more problems with the inflammatory response, than do others. It is a known fact, that inflammation is a cause of fatigue. It also causes our adrenals to remain in overdrive because "cortisol" from the adrenals, is not only the stress hormone but is an anti-inflammatory agent. I feel this is why adrenal fatigue can also be a factor.

Graves' Disease

Thyroid Autoimmunity Resulting in Hyperthyroidism

Statistics estimate that from one to three million Americans suffer from Graves' disease. This thyroid disorder that causes hyperthyroidism (over-active thyroid) is caused by an autoimmune response that sends out antibodies to attack the thyroid gland.

Graves' disease is a type of hyperthyroidism, caused by an autoimmune response in the body. With Graves' disease, a patient will have antibodies sent out by the immune system to attack their thyroid gland. These antibodies attach to the thyroid gland and in response, the gland produces more thyroid hormone and the levels become too high for the body's metabolism to function properly. The sped up metabolism is called "hyperthyroidism" and Graves' disease is the most common cause of an over-functioning thyroid gland.

The antibodies that cause Graves' disease are called "thyroid stimulating immunoglobulin" (TSI). Patients who develop Graves' disease can have several antibodies directed against their thyroid glands. The antibodies cause destruction of the gland, plus swelling and goiter from resulting inflammation. The type of antibody that contributes to the hyper-functioning of the gland, however, is the TSI antibody. These are the ones that help to better diagnose a hyperthyroid patient as having Graves' disease; TSI antibodies are detected in a patient using blood lab testing.

Graves' disease patients can develop nodules on their thyroid glands that contribute to the over-production of thyroid hormone. These nodules are small tumors that begin to develop within the thyroid gland and some of these are what are referred to as "hot nodules", meaning they cause an increase in thyroid hormone production.

Not all nodules that develop in a diseased gland become "hot"; many do not cause the thyroid to become stimulated to over-produce and these are referred to as "cold nodules". Some patients who have multiple nodules that are hot are termed as having a "toxic nodular goiter". If the patient simply has thyroid enlargement or goiter that is characteristic of the disease, it is referred to as "diffuse toxic goiter", which is also another term for Graves' disease.

Treatment for Graves' disease is to slow down thyroid hormone production through the administration of anti-thyroid drugs or removal of the thyroid gland surgically or through radioactive iodine ablation of it (destruction of thyroid tissue). Patients who are first given a trial of anti-thyroid drugs will also be treated with medications to control their symptoms, such as beta-blockers to slow heart rate and reduce the blood pressure and anti-anxiety medications to treat chronic anxiety and/or panic symptoms.

The symptoms of Graves' disease are those of a sped up metabolism. A person with hyperthyroidism, caused by Graves' disease, will experience an overactive metabolism resulting in the following symptoms.

• anxiety and nervousness

• weight loss

• diarrhea

- excessive sweating

- oily skin

- depression

- goiter

- rapid heart rate

- hypertension

- muscle weakness

- tremor

- hair loss

- bone degeneration (osteoporosis)

- increased appetite

Hashimoto's Thyroiditis

Thyroid Autoimmunity Resulting in Hypothyroidism

This type thyroiditis is also autoimmune-caused and results from antibodies attacking the thyroid gland after recognizing it as an intruder in the body and affects at least two million people in the US alone. It is the most common type of thyroiditis in the United States and many other industrialized countries and is also the most common cause of hypothyroidism in the USA.

Over time this attack by auto-antibodies causes damage to the gland and may also cause inflammation and swelling, referred to as "goiter".

Most patients with this type of thyroiditis will experience damage to their thyroid gland over time, causing it to under-function and fail to supply the body with enough thyroid hormone.

The resulting condition as previously mentioned is called "hypothyroidism" which causes symptoms of a slowed bodily metabolism and may include the following.

- fatigue

- depression

- dry skin

- constipation

- joint and muscle aches

- hair loss

- weight gain

- slowed heart rate

- hypotension (low blood pressure)

- fluid retention (edema)

- low libido (sex drive)

- heavy menstrual cycles

Hypothyroidism resulting from Hashimoto's thyroiditis is treated by replacing the missing hormone with a dose of medication containing the proper amount needed.

In some cases, people with Hashimoto's will experience a temporary phase of hyperthyroidism referred to as "Hashitoxicosis". This autoimmune type of thyroiditis is usually life-long in duration.

If symptoms are experienced that suggest the possibility of one of the diseases being present, described in the preceding chapters, it is important that a licensed medical professional be consulted as soon as possible. Early diagnosis can be a key to preventing the progression of these common inflammatory and autoimmune health disorders.

CHAPTER TEN

Osteoarthritis

Arthritis is a word describing joint inflammation in the body, with "arth-" meaning "joint" and "-itis" meaning inflammation. The joints are the places where bones are connected together, so that they move freely, giving mobility to the body and cushioning the joints like shock absorbers to prevent wear and damage to them. Bones can be connected together with "ball and socket", "hinge", "pivot" and "saddle" joints.

According to medical sources that address the subject of arthritis, there are as many as 100 types of arthritic conditions. In the following steps, we will look at the most common type called osteoarthritis.

Osteoarthritis is the most common form of arthritis that exists in the world.

This type of arthritis is caused by wear and tear in the joints of the body, causing deterioration of the cartilage that is found between them. Statistics state that up to 20 million adults are affected by this type of arthritis in the US, and up to 8 million adults are affected in the UK.

Chances for developing osteoarthritis increase after age 40, with a 2% increase for each year following. Seniors have a 50% chance of being diagnosed with this type arthritis by age 65.

The symptoms of osteoarthritis.

People with osteoarthritis will experience pain and stiffness in the affected joints, loss of mobility and mild to moderate inflammation. A single joint may be affected or several joints in the body, but it will usually occur in the joints that are used the most. The joint stiffness in affected areas may be more noticeable upon rising in the morning or at other times when the joints are put back into use after periods of resting them. Weight-bearing joints are the most highly affected in the body.

The diagnosis of osteoarthritis.

Doctors recognize this type of arthritis by checking patients for loss of mobility and pain in joints, due to deterioration in them. An X-ray can further determine the extent of damage that has occurred and, in more sever cases, can also determine if loss of cartilage has resulted in the bones meeting together due to complete lack of joint protection. Joints that are severely affected by osteoarthritis can become fused together over time, causing complete loss of mobility in them.

Treatment for osteoarthritis.

The treatment for this common form of arthritis may consist of lifestyle changes and/or prescribed medications.

A doctor may recommend weight loss in order to reduce pressure on weight-bearing joints, as well as safe well-tolerated exercise to help keep joints mobile. Medications that may be prescribed include over-the-counter and prescription anti-inflammatory drugs, pain medications and, in more severe cases, hydrocortisone injections in the affected joints.

Doctors may sometimes also recommend stress reduction, which can help reduce flares of pain and inflammation. Another recommendation is to use cold or hot compresses on affected joints, which can also help in these areas. Severely affected joints that experience loss of mobility or bone fusion may require corrective surgeries.

It is important to see your doctor if you experience pain, stiffness or a feverish feeling in your joints that may indicate inflammation. Osteoarthritis can be treated more successfully when diagnosed as early as possible.

CHAPTER ELEVEN

Adrenal Insufficiency Basic Facts

While there are other types of adrenal insufficiency that fall under the category of "Addison's disease", the most common type is autoimmune adrenalitis. This article helps us to have better general understanding of this disease. While I'm concentrating on the Addison's type of adrenal insufficiency in this chapter, the symptoms and treatments for all types of adrenal insufficiency are the same or very similar.

Addison's disease is an autoimmune disease affecting the adrenal glands.

Each person has two adrenal glands, which are glands of the endocrine system sitting on top of each kidney in a person's body. These glands are small and shaped like pyramids about the size of a walnut, measuring about 3 x 5 x 1 cm in size. The immune system can mistakenly recognized these glands as intruders and begin to attack them (autoimmune response), slowly destroying them with antibodies (killer cells from the immune system).

This causes the glands to become inadequate in supplying the important adrenal hormones needed by the body, the two major hormones being cortisol and DHEA. Symptoms of Addison's disease appear once the adrenal cortex (the protective outer layer of the gland) has been destroyed by the autoimmune process known as autoimmune adrenalitis.

The symptoms of Addison's disease are those of adrenal insufficiency.

Addison's disease causes adrenal insufficiency, meaning a reduction in adrenal hormone production and output. The two major hormones that become low due to this are cortisol and DHEA.

Cortisol is the "stress hormone" and "anti-inflammatory hormone" that gives the body its ability to handle and recover from stressors and inflammation.

DHEA is a "sex hormone precursor", meaning the hormone that converts into testosterone, estrogen and other hormones needed by the body.

When the adrenal hormones become low, a person may experience fatigue, joint/muscle pain, weight loss and diminished appetite, low blood pressure and hyper-pigmentation (darkening of the skin). If left untreated, people with Addison's disease are at risk of experiencing an adrenal crisis, meaning they will go into shock and possibly coma or death.

Addison's disease is most often diagnosed through blood testing and MRI.

Medical blood lab testing can measure the adrenal hormone levels and if they are found to be low, this can indicate adrenal insufficiency due to Addison's disease. Patients will then usually be tested for adrenal function via an ACTH Stimulation Test.

This test uses the ACTH hormone, which usually comes from a person's own pituitary gland, to stimulate adrenal-cortisol hormone production but, during the test, is administered to the patient by injection.

A patient will have a baseline blood draw taken before the test. After the ACTH hormone injection, they will have two or more additional blood draws taken at 30 minute intervals, and these three blood levels will then be compared. If the two or more additional blood levels of cortisol do not significantly increase above the baseline level, a diagnosis of adrenal insufficiency is confirmed.

Other tests that may be ordered would include an MRI to detect the extent of adrenal gland destruction, and a blood test to detect antibodies that the immune system is directing against the adrenal glands.

Addison's disease is treated by replacing the low adrenal hormone levels.

Once blood tests reveal which adrenal hormones are low, hormone replacement therapy will begin. One of the major hormones called cortisol, which is most commonly low in adrenal insufficiency states, must be replaced with a steroid cortisol substitute called a "glucocorticoid steroid" or a "corticosteroid". Patients will need replacement with this synthetic hormone for the rest of their lives.

Addison's disease patients are also usually required to wear a medical ID bracelet, so that if they experience an adrenal crisis, the person finding them will know that they are treated for Addison's disease and that they may need to have an injection of corticosteroid steroid administered.

There are other causes of adrenal insufficiency, but Addison's disease is the most common, affecting about 1 in 100,000 people according to medical sources. This makes it the least common of the health conditions discussed in the previous chapters.

If one of these disorders is suspected, it is important that a medical professional is consulted with for proper diagnosis and treatment.

CHAPTER TWELVE

A Quick Look at Adrenal Fatigue

Many Doctors only recognize the most severe form of adrenal hypo-function called Addisons' Disease or full blown adrenal insufficiency and they base whether or not a patient has this potentially life-threatening form, via the "ACTH Stimulation Test". The problem is that many people have a less severe form called adrenal fatigue or adrenal exhaustion and though these patients nearly always pass the ACTH Stimulation Test, they still have inadequate adrenal hormone levels that show up clearly on lab tests and though it is not life-threatening, it still causes concerning symptoms that can seriously affect quality of life.

The National Institutes of Health, while studying Chronic Fatigue Syndrome, found "low cortisol" to be a factor in it as well and in one of these studies, they made this statement; *"Doctors have long known that even subtle deficiencies in cortisol can be associated with lethargy and fatigue."*

The "NIAMS" (National Institute of Arthritis and Musculoskeletal and Skin Disease) Division of the National Institutes of Health also recognizes low cortisol in Fibromyalgia. Other studies they've published on the PubMed/National Libraries of Medicine website, also recognize low cortisol in PTSD (Post Traumatic Stress Disorders).

The fact is that adrenal fatigue can be a factor in these and other chronic diseases/syndromes but other times is stress-related or not related to anything specific.

The most important thing, if you feel you may have adrenal fatigue, is to be tested for it because other hormone imbalances and illnesses cause similar symptoms. Some pharmacies are now carrying saliva hormone testing kits, including ones that test adrenal hormones (cortisol), so you may want to check for the availability of these in your area. If they are not available locally, one can order them online using the search term "adrenal hormone saliva test kits".

The passion I have in the area of adrenal fatigue, besides experiencing it myself, as part of CFS and thyroid disease is the fact that far too many studies and reputable organizations recognize it. This includes the "Fibro & Fatigue Centers", located in 15 states that are staffed by Board Certified MDs from just about every field of medicine. This plus the fact that there are U.S. Government health studies that have also concluded that there are low-cortisol syndromes or well established sub-clinical forms of adrenal hypo-function, that could all be referred to under the term; "adrenal fatigue".

There are many supplements that can be self-administered or prescribed by a qualified physician.

These help keep the body and the adrenal glands healthy and strengthened to handle the everyday stress life brings upon all of us. A really good multi-vitamin is always a great idea and there are many good ones available, to choose from. Some major vitamin companies actually manufacture vitamins called "stress formulas" or "stress tabs" and these contain the vitamins and minerals that help the body cope-with and recover from stress.

Vitamin supplements in particular that are very helpful to the adrenal glands include the "B" vitamins – in particular, B-12, B-5 and B-6. Vitamin "C" is also an important vitamin for healthy adrenal function and also serves to help other vitamins absorb properly in the body. Minerals that can help with adrenal function include zinc, selenium and magnesium. There are also adrenal herbal formulas that contain helpful supplements such as "licorice root extract", "Asian ginseng" and "ashwagandha" but these should be researched carefully by anyone who is considering taking them as a short-term or long-term regimen and should also be discussed with your doctor before taking them. Purchasing supplements only from reliable, reputable companies is also wise.

Other natural supplements that can be taken to support the adrenals after observing the aforementioned precautions include "adrenal glandular" (usually beef source) and DHEA, an over-the-counter adrenal hormone.

DHEA also acts as a precursor to sex hormones. All of these supplements can potentially be helpful, but everyone is unique and some supplements work better for some people than they do for others. Sometimes it simply takes a trial of several of these, by a process of elimination, to find the one that eventually helps the most.

CHAPTER THIRTEEN

Mitral Valve Prolapse the Common Heart Murmur

There is a common condition of the heart, that causes concerning symptoms in some patients who have it and it is called "Mitral Valve Prolapse Syndrome". Other patients with the same heart condition do not have symptoms from it and in this case, it is simply called "Mitral Valve Prolapse" (drop the "Syndrome" off the end of the term). Abbreviated, the terms are "MVP" and "MVPS".

In this article, I want to address MVPS, the type that causes symptoms. It is a type of heart murmur, also called a "click murmur" due to a clicking sound that can be heard in the heart, with each beat. The clicking according to medical resources, is caused by the "Mitral Valve Leaflets" becoming somewhat stretched out, so that they are slightly loose or they develop scar tissue on them and become thickened and both of these will cause them to have a slight vibration-effect, when the heart beats, and also causes mild "regurgitation" (blood seepage from the valve) that is picked up as a clicking sound (murmur) on a stethoscope.

Other patients may not have a clicking sound that is as easily heard through a stethoscope but if symptoms they are experiencing, point to MVP, a more sensitive test may be used for detection.

This test is called an Echocardiogram. It uses the same principle as a Sonogram that women who are pregnant get, to monitor the progress of their babies. Sound waves are sent into the area to be observed and they are transmitted onto an image on a screen, so that even the tiniest movement can be seen. This is how patients with more difficult to detect MVP, can be diagnosed or have the condition ruled out as causing their symptoms.

More severe cases of MVP, cause a more severe form of "regurgitation", meaning the blood-leakage from the valves is more significant, when the heart beats. Heart valves of course are supposed to be self-contained, so that blood flows through without leakage from them but with MVP Regurgitation, blood does escape from the valves and this more severe form will sometimes require surgery to correct it however, it is a rare form of MVP.

What are the symptoms of MVP?

A racing heart (tachycardia), heart skips and heart flutters are part of the symptoms but MVPS sufferers, also have fatigue, dizziness, shortness of breath, anxiety symptoms such as panic attacks, "Orthostatic Hypotension" (you also get dizzy upon standing from a seated or lying down position) and sensitivities to chemicals like caffeine, alcohol, tobacco, chocolate and too much sugar. More details about symptoms will follow below.

The chemical sensitivities I mention are triggers, that cause worsening of symptoms in patients with MVPS and the Orthostatic Hypotension, also called "Orthostatic Intolerance", is also classified as a form of "Dysautonomia", meaning you have a slight disregulation of the "Involuntary Nervous System" (INS). Some researchers believe the dysautonomia found in some MVP patients, is what actually causes the syndrome (MVPS) because the Involuntary Nervous System plays a major role in regulating heart rate and blood pressure and when it becomes disregulated due to MVP, this is what causes symptoms, resulting in the syndrome.

In regard to anxiety symptoms found in MVPS, it has been long known that MVP is notorious for causing anxiety attacks and panic attacks and many patients are diagnosed with Anxiety Disorders, due to this underlying medical condition. If these patients can control the symptoms of MVPS, the anxiety symptoms will also be alleviated to a large degree.

Specific signs and symptoms of MVP to look for.

If you notice that you have episodes of skipped heartbeats, heart flutters and flip-flops or rapid heartbeats (tachycardia), this can indicate that you have MVPS.

The irregular heartbeats caused by MVPS are due to slight abnormalities in the mitral valve leaflets, or the supporting valve chords, or both.

These structures allow the leaflet(s) to prolapse (or buckle) back into the left atrium during the heart's contraction-ventricular systole.

While medical research has not concluded definitively what causes the mitral valve to prolapse abnormally in some people, they theorize that it is due to these valve leaflets becoming either thickened or stretched out over time and this causes them to vibrate or quiver slightly. This is why it is referred to as a "click murmur" due to the sound it can sometimes make when the heartbeat is listened to closely with a stethoscope.

If you are experiencing panic attacks and frequent episodes of free-floating anxiety, plus increased depression, this may indicate that you have MVPS.

Anxiety is one of the more frightening symptoms of MVPS because panic attacks are the more common type of anxiety that people with this disorder experience. Medical research is not clear as to how anxiety symptoms are caused by MVPS, but some sources state that it could be due to slightly abnormal electrical impulses in the heart, caused by the abnormal prolapsing of the mitral valve leaflets, which triggers the fight or flight response (adrenaline rush) more frequently or at inappropriate and unexpected times.

While anxiety is listed more commonly for MVPS, depression is also experienced more frequently in these patients.

Patients may find that they more frequently experience both of these emotions simultaneously or they may find that these alternate, so that they are experiencing anxiety at some times and depression at other times.

Dizziness in general and dizziness upon standing from a sitting or lying down position (supine) can indicate that you have MVPS.

The term for getting dizzy upon rising is "orthostatic hypotension" and is a form of "dysautonomia," which is a medical term for an irregular involuntary nervous system. This system of the body, also referred to as the "autonomic nervous system" automatically regulates our involuntary bodily functions, such as heart, respiratory and blood pressure functions.

Certain diseases and disorders, including MVPS, can cause this system of our body to operate abnormally, which results in blood pressure not rising enough upon standing (hypotension) to supply adequate blood circulation to the heart and brain. While this irregular blood pressure upon standing usually only lasts a few seconds, it can also make a person with MVPS; feel faint, dizzy and pressure-type sensations in the head and neck. This dysautonomia aspect may also be the cause of the anxiety symptoms addressed above, according to some medical sources.

If you become short of breath more easily and have less tolerance for exercise and physical exertion, this may indicate you have MVPS.

People with MVPS will find that they become fatigued more easily from exercise and physical exertion and that they become short of breath more easily as well. Tolerance for exercise can become noticeably lowered in people with MVPS when they are experiencing the onset of symptoms not previously experienced.

This syndrome can have an onset (symptom flares) at any age according to medical sources, however the symptoms are more common in women and more commonly found in ages beginning at the mid-teens and older. Some MVPS patients may even find that everyday activities fatigue them more easily and more often than before experiencing the syndrome.

If you have become sensitive to caffeine, chocolate, alcohol, excess sugar and stimulants, this may indicate you have MVPS.

People who are experiencing MVPS find that they have unpleasant aftereffects from foods and drinks containing stimulant-type chemicals. Tobacco use can also cause symptom flares. These people will find that overindulgence of these chemicals or that even small to moderate amounts of any of these stimulants can cause symptom reactions.

Even an extra cup of coffee or a chocolate bar can cause their heart to skip beats or flutter and can also trigger anxiety attacks, depression and fatigue more easily. We could also add "stress" to this category because stress is stimulating and a necessary mechanism in our daily lives however, stress levels that are excessive or prolonged can cause the same symptom flares in MVPS patients that these other stimulants can.

While a patient will notice the symptoms we've addressed above, before they suspect that MVPS could be the cause, these are simply observations that should prompt a visit to their licensed physician. Once a patient has described their symptoms to their doctor, he can perform a physical, including listening closely to the patient's heart.

He may detect a heart murmur by stethoscope but in many cases, MVP cannot be detected unless the patient is sent (referred) to a cardiologist (heart specialist) for a test called an "echocardiogram." This test is similar to ultrasound in that it uses very sensitive sound waves, transmitted onto a screen, so that the function of the heart can be monitored very clearly. If a patient has Mitral Valve Prolapse, the condition will be detected and definitively diagnosed using this diagnostic test.

Treatments for MVP.

In more severe cases of MVP, a patient can experience what is called "regurgitation" in the heart, meaning that there may be some back-flow of blood into the atrium due to the prolapse. This form of MVP is very rare but can require surgery if it is severe enough.

For most patients with MVP, the treatment sometimes is simply taking a beta-blocker for rapid heart rate and blood pressure fluctuations. In some patients, their doctor may simply have them follow a regimen of improved diet, excluding stimulants and regular exercise, plus stress reduction. The diet aspect would be, to avoid stimulants in your diet (caffeine, alcohol, tobacco, stress and chocolate) that can be triggers for MVPS symptoms.

Also a healthy diet with lots of fruits and vegetables is always a good idea. Also a good multi-vitamin helps the body's systems operate at a more optimal level. Exercise can be of more benefit than any other single factor but a patient must pace their self and only exercise at their tolerance-level, then increase that level as they are able.

Walking is a great way to begin an exercise program and even if you only increase the distance and/or briskness of your walk over time, the benefits can be tremendous.

MVP patients are sometimes also found to be low in magnesium; a mineral the body needs for proper heart function. In cases of low magnesium, the patient simply takes a supplement to get the mineral back to the proper level.

CHAPTER FOURTEEN

CFS and Fibromyalgia – The Syndromes of Fatigue and Muscle Pain

Chronic Fatigue Syndrome and Fibromyalgia affect millions of Americans and many millions more worldwide. The Debilitating fatigue and joint/muscle pain these syndromes cause can seriously reduce the quality-of-life for those who experience them. Aspects of these illnesses can include the following.

• Viral, fungal and bacterial components

• hormonal and nutritional deficiencies

• adrenal fatigue (low cortisol and/or DHEA levels)

Chronic Fatigue Syndrome and Fibromyalgia are real illnesses recognized by the U.S. National Institutes of Health and other World Health Organizations. While they are separately recognized illnesses, they have 75% crossover similarities. Because of this, many medical sources involved in research regarding these syndromes, believe they may indeed be the same illness that presents in one of two different variations.

Since many symptoms of CFS and Fibromyalgia are in-common with both syndromes, the symptom list that follows will be an equal possibility for being experienced with both syndromes.

With the two major characteristic symptoms that distinguish between the two syndromes being "fatigue" (CFS) and "body pain" (Fibromyalgia). Both can be present in each illness but if one or the other is prominent, this helps to distinguish between them.

Some basic symptoms common for both syndromes include the following:

• Fatigue (ongoing and following exertion)

• Joint/muscle aches & tender points (with the absence of redness or swelling of joints)

• Neurological symptoms (i.e. headaches, tremors, dizziness and sensory changes)

• Emotional symptoms (i.e. anxiety and/or depression)

• Cognitive problems (i.e. difficulty concentrating and short-term memory loss)

These two syndromes mimic the symptoms of many other disorders as well, including those addressed in the preceding chapters. This can make diagnosis a difficult and sometimes lengthy process because all other medical conditions must be ruled-out before CFS and/or Fibromyalgia are definitively identified.

Treatments for these illnesses, consists of targeting the symptoms to provide relief of them and to restore quality of life to the patient.

Correcting any hormone or nutritional deficiencies is very important in this process, as well as providing pain relief and increasing low energy levels when possible. Depending on the type of MD or other category of physician that administers treatment (i.e. Osteopath, Endocrinologist, Neurologist or Naturopath), a patient may be prescribed either pharmaceutical drugs or natural supplements or a combination of both. Patients may also be referred to a mental health professional for emotional symptoms if psychotropic drugs alone do not adequately provide relief of them (i.e. SSRI antidepressants and benzodiazepines).

Less-common treatments for CFS and Fibromyalgia include use of anti-viral drugs and those that boost immune system function. In some cases, these illnesses will resolve over time even when treatments are not being administered and the course of them can vary from being 2 years in length, 5 years or even lifelong. The age of patients, their overall health status and their lifestyle habits can all be factors in the course and severity of these syndromes.

When the symptoms of any of the illnesses described in this chapter and the preceding ones, are being experienced, it is important to see a qualified medical professional for further evaluation. Treatments are available for these health disorders but due to the potential damaging effects of delayed treatment, early diagnosis of them is very important.

It is my hope that I have provided an informative general description that can help readers to identify illnesses that can potentially affect them or their family members. It is however important to remember that a licensed physician is required to rule-out or to definitively diagnose medical illnesses.

(END)